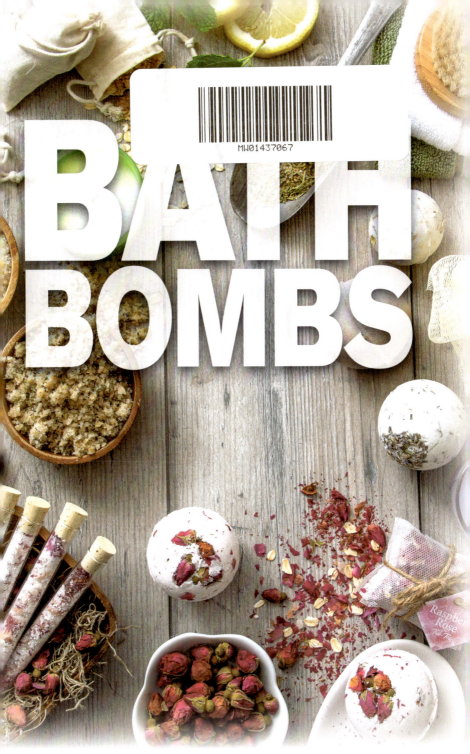

BATH BOMBS

MW01437067

Copyright © 2018 CQ Products
All rights reserved.
No part of this book may be reproduced or transmitted in any form
or by any means, electronic or mechanical, including photocopying,
recording or by any information storage and retrieval system,
without permission in writing from the publisher.

ISBN-13: 978-1-56383-579-7
Item #2621

Printed in the USA

www.cqbookstore.com

<u>Distributed By:</u>

gifts@cqbookstore.com

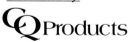

507 Industrial Street
Waverly, IA 50677

 CQ Products

 CQ Products

 @cqproducts

 @cqproducts

Turn every day into *Spa Day!*

Relaxation is the name of the game on a spa day. Follow these tips to ensure the process of making your homemade bath bombs, salts, scrubs, and teas is just as relaxing as using them.

Know Your Ingredients: It's always best to be familiar with ingredients before adding them to your bath. It's possible some allergies or irritation could occur depending on your skin sensitivities. It's important to take the time to find which ingredients work best with your skin.

Soak Safely: Many of the recipes in this book include natural oils to help moisturize and soften skin. While these oils have amazing benefits, they can leave your tub a little on the slippery side. We recommend using a shower mat and being extra careful while getting in and out of the tub. And remember, none of these recipes are edible, no matter how yummy they smell!

Easy Cleanup: It's best to rinse the tub immediately after use for easy cleanup. This will wash away any residual oils, dyes, or particles left over from the bath.

Get Creative: Use the recipes in this book as guides, but don't be afraid to customize them to your liking! Many recipes call for colorants or embellishments to dress them up for gifting, but these are always optional. Your creations can be as simple or complex as you want them to be. Once you master the basics, you'll be concocting your own recipes in no time!

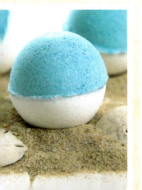
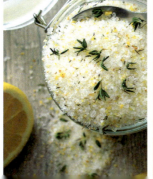
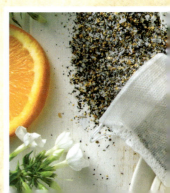

Bath Bombs

 A bath bomb base *consists of four simple ingredients.*

Baking Soda *is part of the chemical reaction that gives bath bombs their fizz.*

Citric Acid *is the other half of the reaction. It can be found online or in the canning section of most stores.*

Cornstarch *hardens the bath bomb and leaves skin silky smooth.*

Liquid *is needed to bind bath bombs together. Rubbing alcohol works well because it evaporates quickly.*

 It's the **add-ins** *that make each recipe unique!*

Fragrances *can be added with essential oils, dried herbs, spices, or cosmetic-grade fragrance oils.*

Carrier Oils *moisturize skin and disperse essential oils. Olive and coconut are great choices.*

Epsom Salt *is believed to soothe muscle pain.*

Powdered Milk *softens and moisturizes skin.*

Color *can be added with food coloring. When in doubt, use less than you think you'll need.*

Molds *for bath bombs are sold online, but muffin tins, Easter eggs, and ice cube trays also work well.*

Follow the basic instructions below when making bath bombs. Each recipe will make 3 to 4 (2½") bath bombs.

1 In a large bowl, whisk together the dry ingredients.

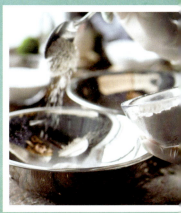

2 In a small bowl, combine the liquid ingredients *(excluding food coloring)*.

3 Slowly pour the liquid mixture into the dry mixture, whisking as you go. Slow down if the mixture begins to fizz. *Note: If creating multicolored layers, divide this mixture between multiple bowls and dye each the desired color.*

4 Mix in any food coloring.

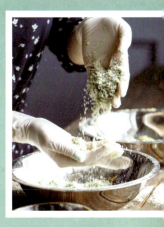

5 With a spray bottle, spritz the mixture with rubbing alcohol and use your hands to combine, spritzing as needed, until it begins to retain its shape when packed in your hands. Be careful not to add too much liquid, as this can cause bath bombs to prematurely fizz.

6 Add any embellishments to the molds and tightly pack in the mixture. If using spherical molds, slightly overfill each half and firmly press them together for 30 seconds.

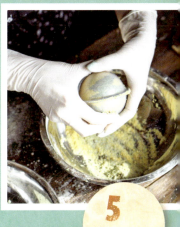

7 Remove the top of the mold and let dry overnight before removing the bottom mold.

8 Let dry for an additional 24 hours before wrapping with plastic or storing in an airtight container.

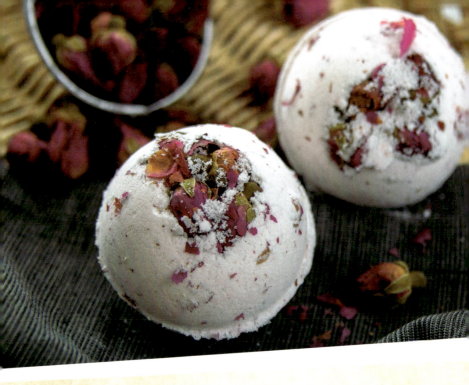

Pink Rose

- 1 C. baking soda
- ½ C. citric acid
- ¼ C. cornstarch
- ¼ C. powdered milk
- ¼ C. dried rose buds, crushed
- 2 tsp. coconut oil, melted
- 5 drops geranium essential oil
- 15 drops rose essential oil
- Red food coloring (optional)
- Rubbing alcohol in a spray bottle
- Extra dried rose buds for embellishment (optional)
- Bath bomb molds

Follow the basic bath bomb instructions on page 5.

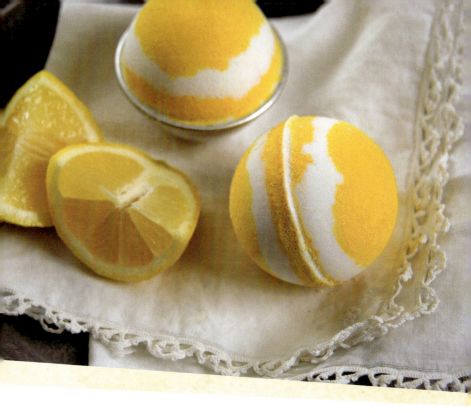

Lemon Drop

1 C. baking soda

½ C. cornstarch

½ C. citric acid

2 tsp. coconut oil, melted

15 drops lemongrass
   essential oil

¼ tsp. pure vanilla extract

Yellow food coloring
   (optional)

Rubbing alcohol
   in a spray bottle

Bath bomb molds

Follow the basic bath bomb instructions on page 5.

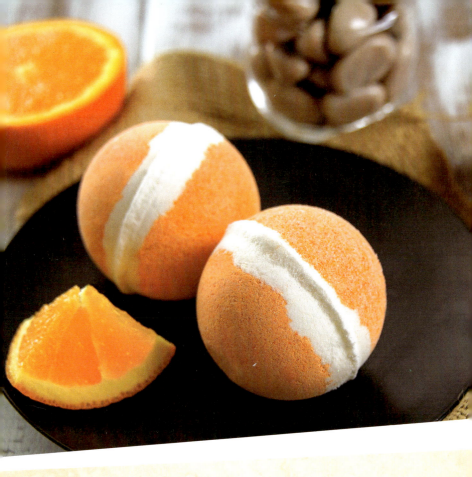

Orange Creamsicle

1 C. baking soda

½ C. citric acid

¼ C. powdered milk

¼ C. cornstarch

2 tsp. olive oil

15 drops sweet orange
essential oil

¼ tsp. pure vanilla extract

Orange food coloring
(optional)

Rubbing alcohol
in a spray bottle

Bath bomb molds

1. In a large bowl, whisk together the baking soda, citric acid, powdered milk, and cornstarch.

2. In a small bowl, mix together the olive oil, essential oil, and extract.

3. Slowly pour the oil mixture into the bowl of dry ingredients, whisking as you go. Slow down if the mixture begins to fizz.

4. Split this mixture evenly between two bowls.

5. Mix the food coloring into the first bowl.

6. Spritz the first bowl with rubbing alcohol and use your hands to combine, spritzing as needed, until it begins to retain its shape when packed in your hands. Repeat this process for the second bowl.

7. Layer the orange and white mixtures into the molds. If using spherical molds, slightly overfill each half and firmly press them together for 30 seconds.

8. Remove the top of the mold and let dry overnight before removing the bottom.

9. Let the bath bombs dry for an additional 24 hours before wrapping with plastic or storing in an airtight container.

Gifting

Put a loofa in the bottom of a wide-mouth Mason jar and top with homemade bath bombs. Add a hang tag to complete the gift!

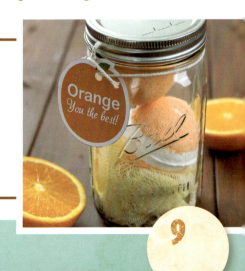

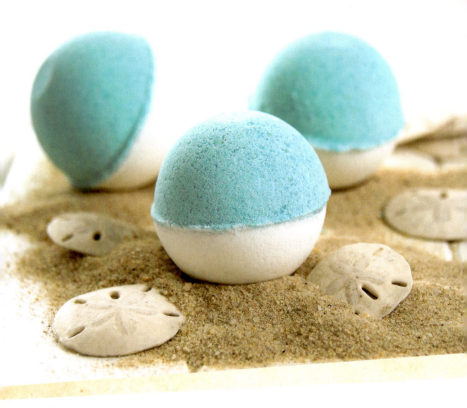

Ocean Breeze

1 C. baking soda

½ C. citric acid

¼ C. cornstarch

¼ C. Epsom salt

2 tsp. coconut oil, melted

6 drops lavender
   essential oil

6 drops lime essential oil

3 drops wintergreen
   essential oil

Blue food coloring
   (optional)

Rubbing alcohol
   in a spray bottle

Bath bomb molds

Follow the basic bath bomb instructions on page 5.

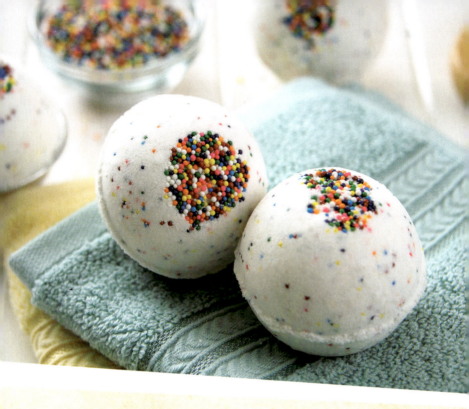

Funfetti

1 C. baking soda

½ C. citric acid

¼ C. cornstarch

¼ C. powdered milk

¼ C. rainbow sprinkles

2 tsp. coconut oil, melted

¼ tsp. pure almond extract

¼ tsp. pure vanilla extract

Rubbing alcohol in a spray bottle

Extra rainbow sprinkles for embellishment (optional)

Bath bomb molds

Follow the basic bath bomb instructions on page 5.

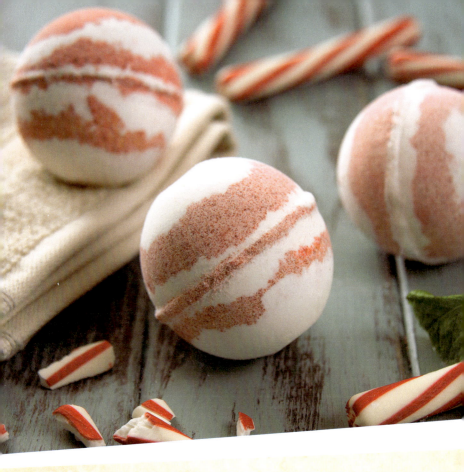

Candy Cane

1 C. baking soda

½ C. citric acid

½ C. cornstarch

2 tsp. coconut oil, melted

15 drops peppermint
   essential oil

¼ tsp. pure vanilla extract

Red food coloring (optional)

Rubbing alcohol
   in a spray bottle

Bath bomb molds

1. In a large bowl, whisk together the baking soda, citric acid, and cornstarch.

2. In a small bowl, mix together the coconut oil, essential oil, and extract.

3. Slowly add the liquid mixture to the dry mixture, whisking as you go. Slow down if the mixture begins to fizz.

4. Split this mixture evenly between two bowls.

5. Mix the food coloring into the first bowl.

6. Spritz the first bowl with rubbing alcohol and combine, spritzing as needed, until it begins to retain its shape when packed in your hands. Repeat this process for the second bowl.

7. Layer the mixtures into the molds to create an alternating pattern. If using spherical molds, slightly overfill each half and firmly press them together for 30 seconds.

8. Remove the top of the mold and let dry overnight before removing the bottom.

9. Let the bath bombs dry for an additional 24 hours before wrapping with plastic or storing in an airtight container.

Gifting

Wrap bath bombs in plastic wrap and then a square of fabric. Twist each end of the fabric and fasten with string to create a candy-inspired look.

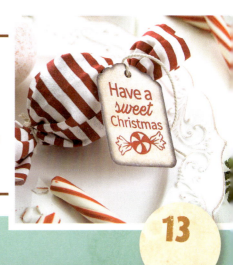

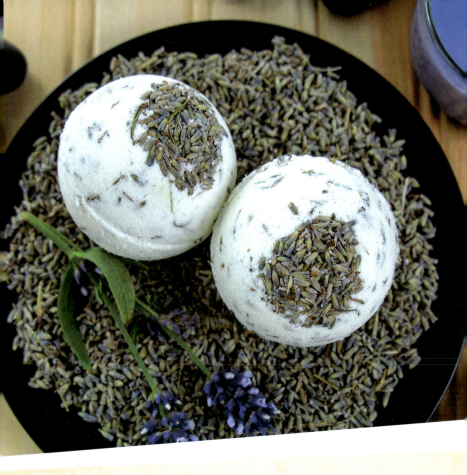

Lovely Lavender

1 C. baking soda

¼ C. cornstarch

½ C. citric acid

¼ C. Epsom salt

2 tsp. dried lavender buds

2 tsp. olive oil

15 drops lavender
essential oil

Rubbing alcohol
in a spray bottle

Extra lavender buds for
embellishment (optional)

Bath bomb molds

1. In a large bowl, whisk together the baking soda, cornstarch, citric acid, Epsom salt, and dried lavender buds.

2. In a small bowl, combine the olive oil and lavender essential oil.

3. Slowly pour the liquid mixture into the dry mixture, whisking as you go. Slow down if the mixture begins to fizz.

4. Spritz the mixture with rubbing alcohol and use your hands to combine, spritzing as needed, until it begins to retain its shape when packed in your hands. Be careful not to add too much liquid, as this can cause bath bombs to prematurely fizz.

5. Sprinkle a few lavender buds into the bottom of each mold.

6. Tightly pack the mixture into the molds. If using spherical molds, slightly overfill each half and firmly press them together for 30 seconds.

7. Remove the top half of the mold and let dry overnight before removing the bottom mold.

8. Let the bath bombs dry for an additional 24 hours before wrapping with plastic or storing in an airtight container

Gifting

Wrap a bath bomb in plastic wrap and then with a square of fabric. Cinch shut with twine and add a tag to complete the gift.

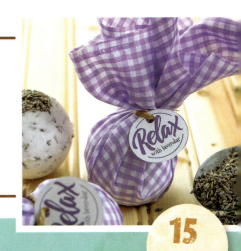

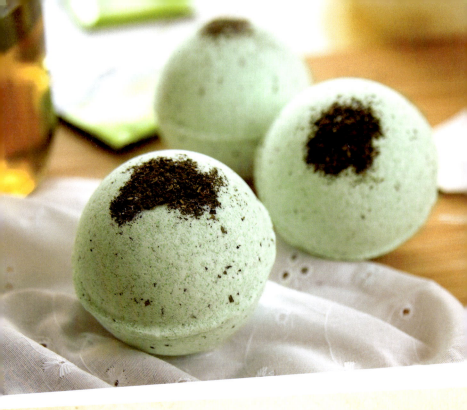

Green Tea

1 C. baking soda

½ C. cornstarch

½ C. citric acid

The contents of
    1 green teabag

4 drops lemongrass
    essential oil

2 tsp. coconut oil, melted

Green food coloring
    (optional)

Rubbing alcohol
    in a spray bottle

Extra green tea for
    embellishment
    (optional)

Bath bomb molds

Follow the basic bath bomb instructions on page 5.

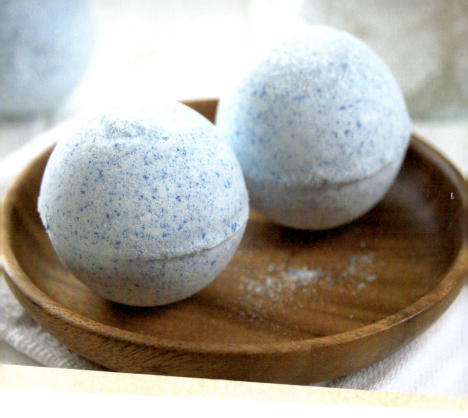

Double Mint

- 1 C. baking soda
- ½ C. citric acid
- ½ C. cornstarch
- 2 tsp. coconut oil, melted
- 8 drops peppermint essential oil
- 12 drops wintergreen essential oil

- Blue food coloring (optional)
- Rubbing alcohol in a spray bottle
- Sugar crystals for embellishment (optional)
- Bath bomb molds

Follow the basic bath bomb instructions on page 5.

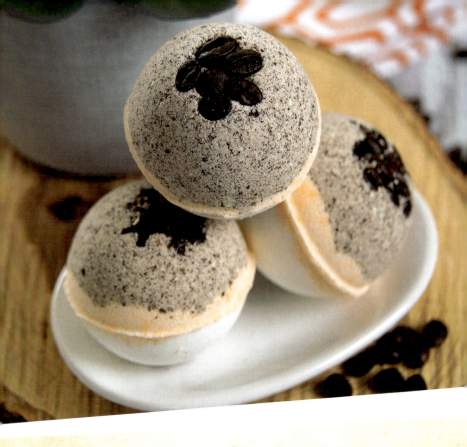

Pumpkin Spice Latte

- 1 C. baking soda
- ½ C. citric acid
- ½ C. cornstarch
- 2 tsp. coconut oil, melted
- 2 drops cinnamon essential oil
- 1 tsp. pumpkin pie spice
- ½ tsp. ground cinnamon

- 2 tsp. instant coffee granules
- Orange food coloring (optional)
- Rubbing alcohol in a spray bottle
- Whole coffee beans for embellishment (optional)
- Bath bomb molds

1. In a large bowl, whisk together the baking soda, citric acid, and cornstarch.

2. In a small bowl, mix together the coconut oil and essential oil

3. Slowly pour the liquid mixture into the dry mixture, whisking as you go.

4. Split this mixture evenly between three bowls.

5. Mix the pumpkin pie spice, cinnamon, and instant coffee into the first bowl.

6. Mix orange food coloring into the second bowl.

7. Spritz the first mixture with rubbing alcohol and combine, spritzing as needed, until it begins to retain its shape when packed in your hands. Repeat this process for all three mixtures.

8. Add a few coffee beans to the bottom of each mold and layer in the mixtures. Slightly overfill the molds and firmly press together for 30 seconds.

9. Remove the top mold and let dry overnight before removing the bottom mold. Let dry for an additional 24 hours before wrapping with plastic or storing in an airtight container.

Gifting

For a professional wrap, lay plastic wrap over the bath bomb, gather in the back, and twist until taut. Secure with tape and cut away the excess.

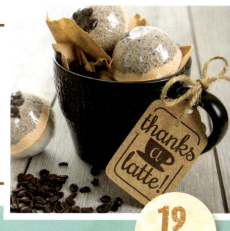

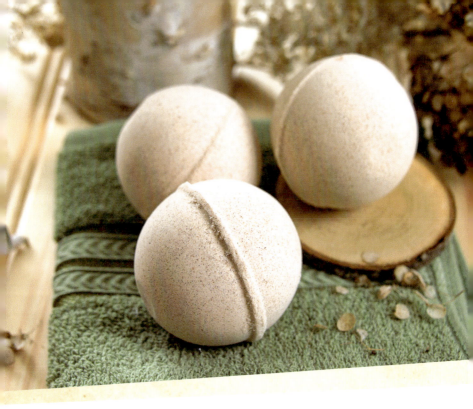

Warm Woods

1 C. baking soda

½ C. citric acid

½ C. cornstarch

1 tsp. ground cinnamon

2 tsp. olive oil

10 drops vetiver
essential oil

5 drops cedar essential oil

5 drops sandalwood
essential oil

Rubbing alcohol
in a spray bottle

Bath bomb molds

Follow the basic bath bomb instructions on page 5.

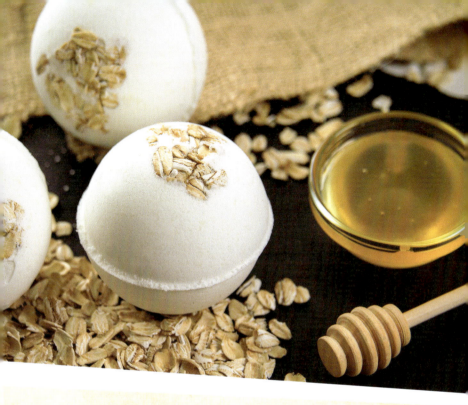

Milk & Honey

1 C. baking soda

½ C. citric acid

¼ C. powdered milk

¼ C. cornstarch

2 tsp. olive oil

¼ tsp. pure vanilla extract

1 T. honey, warmed

Rubbing alcohol
in a spray bottle

Old-fashioned oats
for embellishment
(optional)

Bath bomb molds

Follow the basic bath bomb instructions on page 5.

Bath Salts

Bath salts include a variety of ingredients that can be mixed and matched to create unique recipes!

Epsom Salt is believed to soothe muscle pain and relieve tension.

Baking Soda helps alleviate irritation and soften skin.

Salt is full of beneficial minerals that rehydrate and improve skin texture. Sea salt, dead sea salt, and Himalayan pink salt are all great choices.

Powdered Milk contains fats and proteins that help hydrate skin and retain moisture.

Fragrance can be added with essential oils, dried herbs, spices, teas, or cosmetic-grade fragrance oils.

Color can be added with food coloring. When in doubt, use less than you think you'll need.

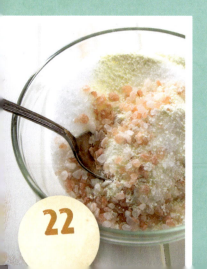

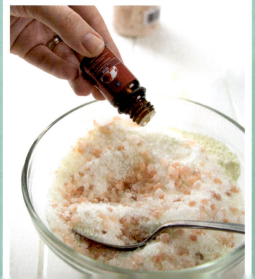

Follow the basic instructions below when making bath salts. Each recipe will make enough bath salts for approximately 12 baths.

1 Whisk together the dry ingredients.

2 Drop in any essential oils, extracts, or food coloring and mix until they're evenly dispersed throughout the mixture. Be sure to break up any clumps that may have formed.

3 Add any dried flowers, spices, or herbs and gently combine.

4 If the mixture seems damp, spread on a sheet pan and let dry for a couple of hours.

5 Store the bath salts in an airtight container.

How to use bath salts:

Add 3-4 tablespoons of bath salts to a warm bath and enjoy! Rinse the tub after use for easy cleanup.

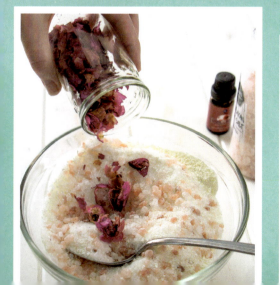

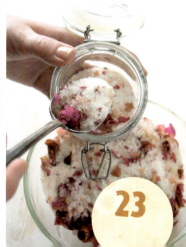

23

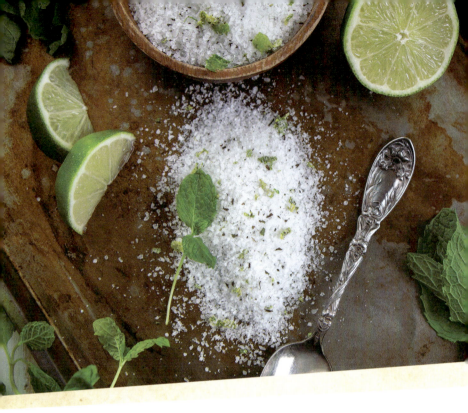

Mojito

2 C. Epsom salt

1 C. coarse sea salt

10 drops peppermint essential oil

10 drops lime essential oil

Zest of 1 lime

1 T. dried mint

Follow the basic bath salt instructions on page 23.

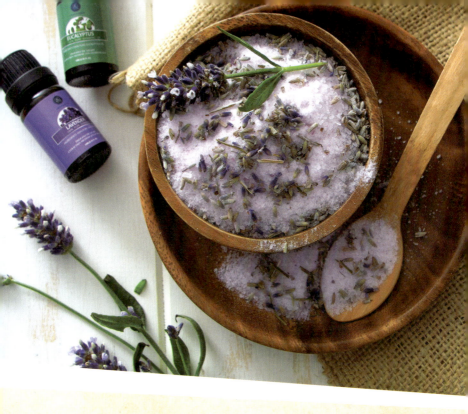

Eucalyptus Lavender

2 C. Epsom salt

½ C. coarse sea salt

½ C. baking soda

10 drops lavender essential oil

10 drops eucalyptus essential oil

¼ C. dried lavender buds

Follow the basic bath salt instructions on page 23.

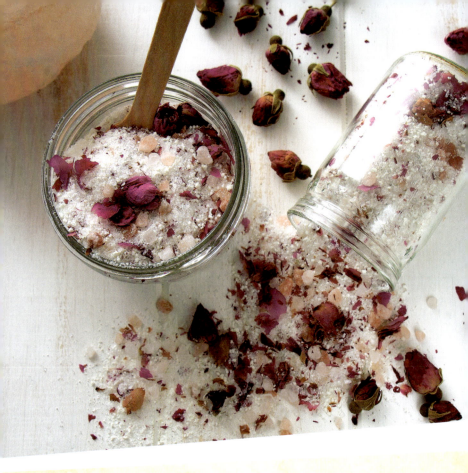

Rose Milk

1 C. Epsom salt

½ C. coarse sea salt

½ C. Himalayan pink salt

1 C. powdered milk

15 drops rose essential oil

5 drops geranium essential oil

3 drops lavender essential oil

½ C. dried rose buds

1. Whisk together the Epsom salt, coarse sea salt, Himalayan pink salt, and powdered milk.

2. Drop in the essential oils and stir until they are evenly dispersed throughout the mixture. Be sure to break up any clumps that may have formed.

3. Remove the hard, green bases from the rose buds and crush the buds into smaller pieces.

4. Gently stir the crushed rose buds into the salt mixture.

5. Transfer the bath salts into an airtight container for storage.

Gifting

Fill glass test tubes with homemade bath salts and top with a cork. Each test tube will be perfectly portioned for a bath!

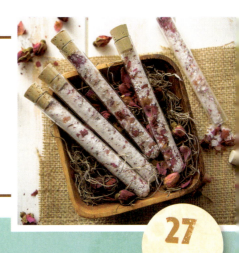

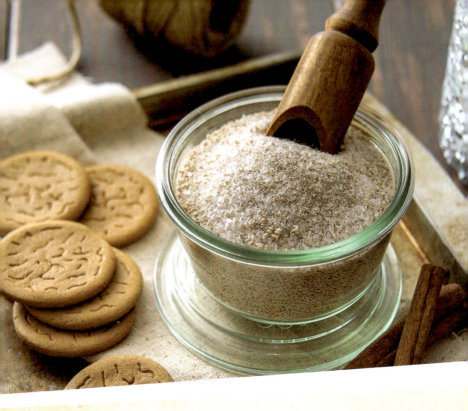

Gingerbread

2½ C. Epsom salt

½ C. powdered milk

10 drops cinnamon essential oil

½ tsp. pure vanilla extract

½ tsp. ground cinnamon

½ tsp. ground ginger

½ tsp. ground allspice

Follow the basic bath salt instructions on page 23.

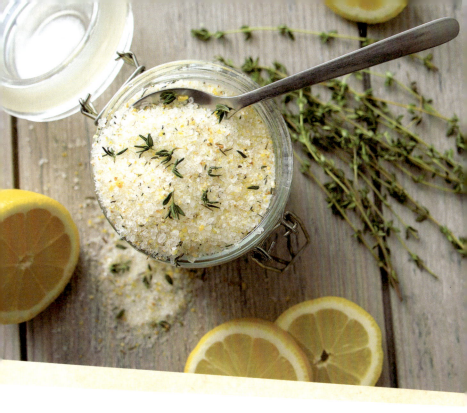

Lemon Thyme

2 C. Epsom salt

1 C. coarse sea salt

10 drops lemongrass
   essential oil

Yellow food coloring
(optional)

2 tsp. dried thyme

1 tsp. dried lemon peel

Follow the basic bath salt instructions on page 23.

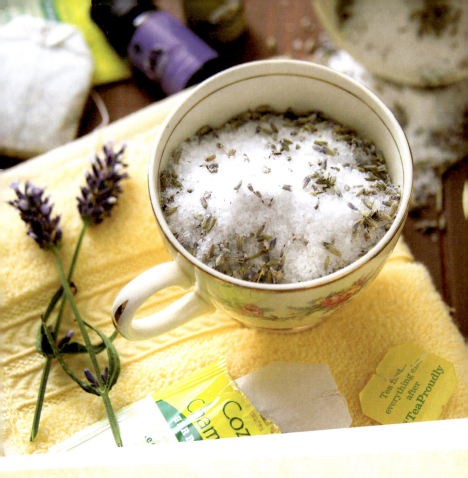

Lavender Chamomile

2 C. Epsom salt

1 C. coarse sea salt

15 drops lavender
essential oil

5 drops chamomile
essential oil

The contents of
3 chamomile teabags

¼ C. dried lavender buds

1. Whisk together the Epsom salt and coarse sea salt.

2. Drop in the essential oils and stir until they are evenly dispersed throughout the mixture. Be sure to break up any clumps that may have formed.

3. Cut open the chamomile teabags and mix the contents into the salt mixture.

4. Add the lavender buds and gently stir until evenly combined.

5. Transfer the bath salts into an airtight container for storage.

Gifting

Funnel your homemade salts into a unique bottle and add a hang tag to complete the gift!

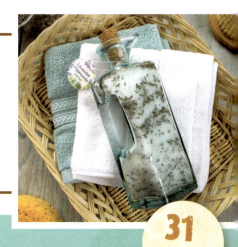

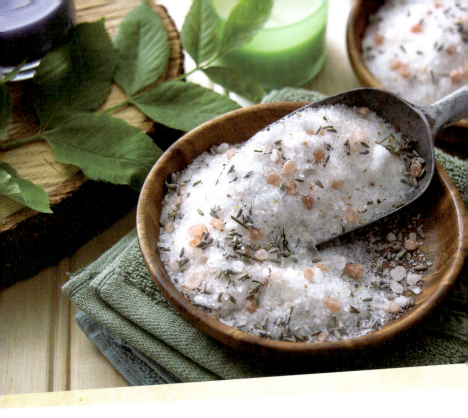

Mountain Air

2 C. Epsom salt

½ C. coarse sea salt

½ C. Himalayan pink salt

10 drops cedar
    essential oil

5 drops vetiver
    essential oil

3 drops sweet orange
    essential oil

1 tsp. dried orange peel

1 T. dried lavender buds

Follow the basic bath salt instructions on page 23.

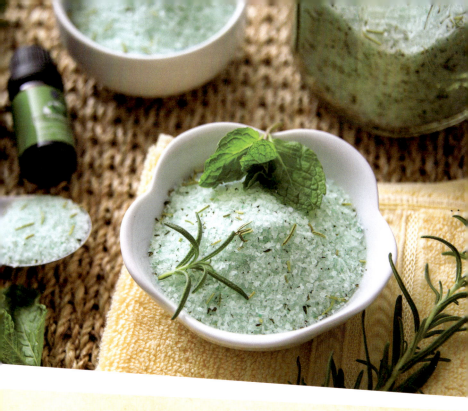

Rosemary Mint

2 C. Epsom salt

1 C. coarse sea salt

15 drops peppermint essential oil

5 drops rosemary essential oil

Green food coloring (optional)

2 tsp. dried mint

1 tsp. dried rosemary

Follow the basic bath salt instructions on page 23.

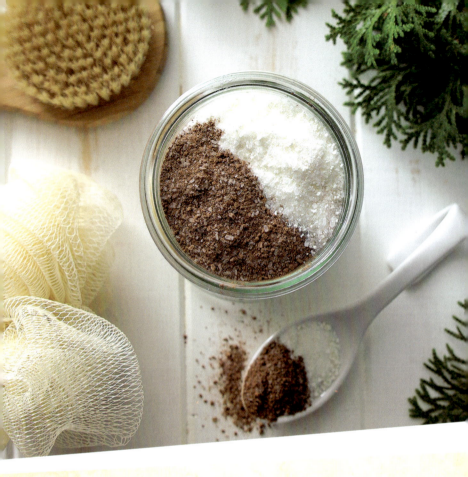

Soothing Hot Cocoa

2½ C. Epsom salt

½ C. powdered milk

1 T. unsweetened cocoa
powder

5 drops peppermint
essential oil

½ tsp. pure vanilla extract

1. In a large bowl, whisk together the Epsom salt and powdered milk.

2. Split this mixture evenly between two bowls.

3. Add the cocoa powder to the first bowl and whisk until evenly combined.

4. Add the peppermint essential oil and vanilla extract to the second bowl and stir until evenly dispersed. Be sure to break up any clumps that may have formed.

5. Combine the mixtures and store in an airtight container, or for a decorative touch, keep the mixtures separate and layer them into a clear container to create an alternating pattern.

Gifting

For a unique holiday gift, funnel homemade bath salts into a clear Christmas ornament to create alternating layers.

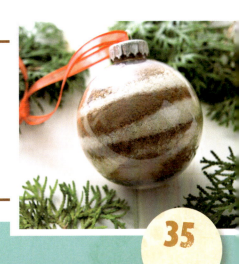

Body Scrubs

Basic scrubs consist of an exfoliant, a nourishing liquid, and some extra add-ins to make each recipe unique.

Exfoliants

Salt, sugar, ground coffee, and oatmeal are all great exfoliant options. Salt tends to be the most abrasive and does a great job at smoothing rougher skin. Sugar, ground coffee, and oatmeal are less abrasive and work well as gentle exfoliants for sensitive skin types.

Liquids

Natural oils such as coconut, olive, and almond help moisturize and soften the skin. Honey contains natural anti-bacterial and anti-inflammatory properties that make it a great addition to scrubs.

Add-ins

Extra add-ins are what make each scrub unique. Adding essential oils, dried flowers, herbs, spices, or zests are all great ways to jazz up a scrub.

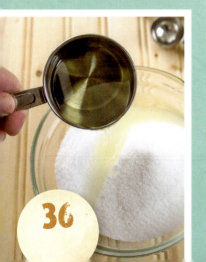

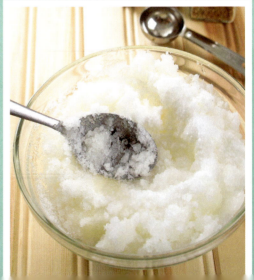

Follow the basic instructions below when making body scrubs. Each scrub recipe will make approximately 2½ cups of scrub.

1 Whisk together the dry ingredients.

2 Slowly add the oil or honey to the dry ingredients, stirring as you go. You want a consistency that can be easily scooped with your hands.

3 Mix in any essential oils, extracts, or food coloring.

4 Add any dried herbs, flowers, zests, or spices and gently mix again.

5 Store in an airtight container in a cool, dark place.

Note: The shelf life of a scrub varies depending on the ingredients.

How to use body scrubs:

Gently apply a small amount of scrub to damp skin in a circular motion and rinse off with warm water. Don't exfoliate more than 2-3 times a week as this can over-exfoliate and damage skin.

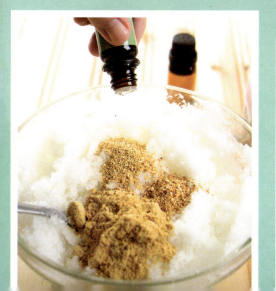

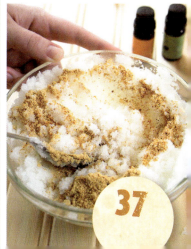

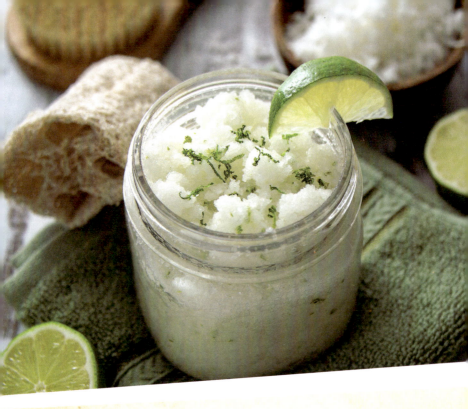

Coconut Lime

1 C. pure cane sugar

1 C. coarse sea salt

¼ C. coconut oil, melted

¼ C. olive oil

5 drops lime essential oil

Zest of 1 lime

Follow the basic scrub instructions on page 37. Store in an airtight container for up to 2 months.

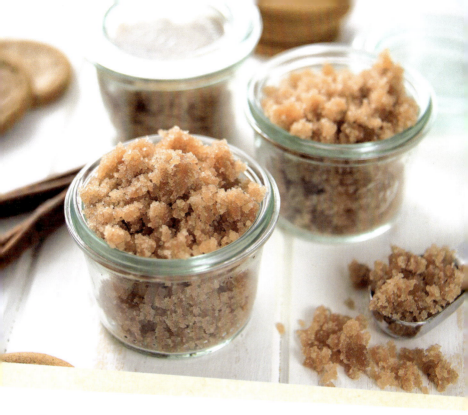

Cookie Dough

½ C. brown sugar

1½ C. pure cane sugar

1 tsp. unsweetened cocoa powder

½ C. olive oil

½ tsp. pure vanilla extract

Follow the basic scrub instructions on page 37. Store in an airtight container for up to 2 months.

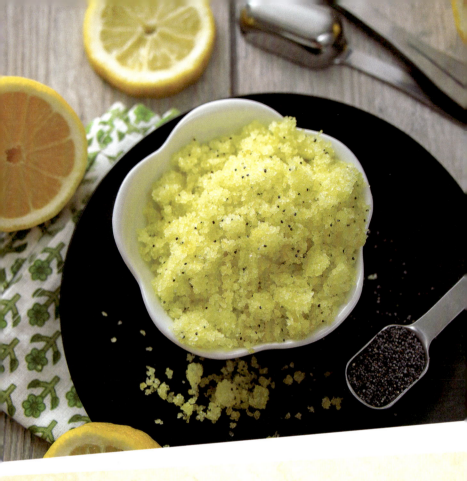

Lemon Poppy Seed

1 C. Epsom salt

1 C. pure cane sugar

½ C. olive oil

10 drops lemongrass
essential oil

½ tsp. pure vanilla extract

Yellow food coloring
(optional)

1 T. poppy seeds

1. Whisk together the Epsom salt and sugar.

2. In a separate bowl, stir together the olive oil, essential oil, extract, and food coloring.

3. Slowly pour the oil mixture into the dry ingredients, stirring as you go. Be sure to break up any clumps that may have formed.

4. Add the poppy seeds to the mixture and mix until evenly dispersed throughout the mixture.

5. Transfer the scrub into an airtight container.

6. Store in a cool, dark place for up to 2 months.

Gifting

Transfer the homemade scrub into a swing-top jar. Add a gift tag and a salt scoop for a decorative touch!

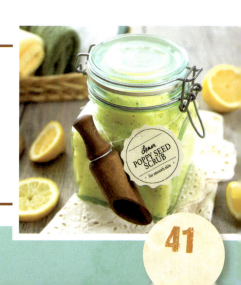

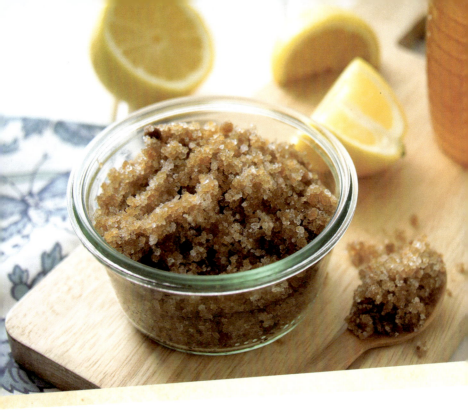

Honey Lemon

1 C. brown sugar

1 C. coarse sea salt

¼ C. honey

¼ C. olive oil

10 drops lemongrass
essential oil

Follow the basic scrub instructions on page 37. Store in
an airtight container for up to 2 months.

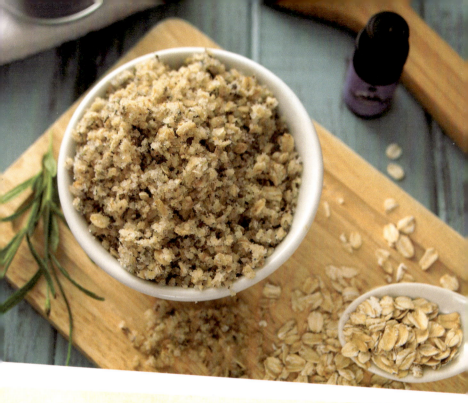

Lavender Oats

1 C. old-fashioned oats

1 C. pure cane sugar

½ C. olive oil

10 drops lavender essential oil

½ tsp. pure vanilla extract

3 T. dried lavender buds

Place the oats in a food processor and pulse until coarsely ground. Follow the basic scrub instructions on page 37. Store in the refrigerator for up to 3 weeks.

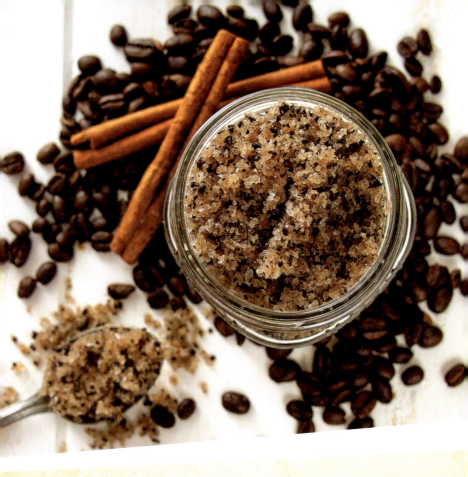

Spiced Mocha

½ C. pure cane sugar

1 C. Epsom salt

½ C. coarse sea salt

¼ C. ground coffee

½ tsp. ground cinnamon

1 T. unsweetened cocoa powder

½ C. olive oil

2 drops cinnamon essential oil

½ tsp. pure vanilla extract

1 Whisk together the sugar, Epsom salt, sea salt, ground coffee, cinnamon, and cocoa powder.

2 In a separate bowl, stir together the olive oil, essential oil, and extract.

3 Slowly pour the oil mixture into the dry mixture, stirring until the oil is evenly dispersed throughout the mixture. Be sure to break up any large clumps that may have formed.

4 Transfer the scrub into an airtight container.

5 Store the scrub in a cool, dark place for up to 4 weeks.

Gifting

Transfer the scrub into a spice jar. Tie a spoon and a gift tag to the jar to complete the gift!

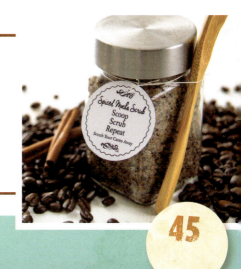

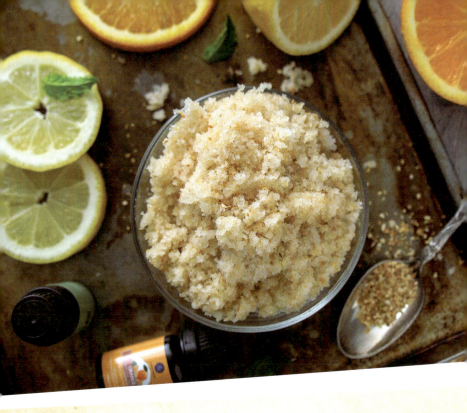

Citrus Ginger

1 C. pure cane sugar

1 C. Epsom salt

½ C. olive oil

6 drops sweet orange
essential oil

4 drops lemongrass
essential oil

2 T. ground ginger

1 tsp. dried lemon peel

1 tsp. dried orange peel

Follow the basic scrub instructions on page 37. Store in an airtight container for up to 2 months.

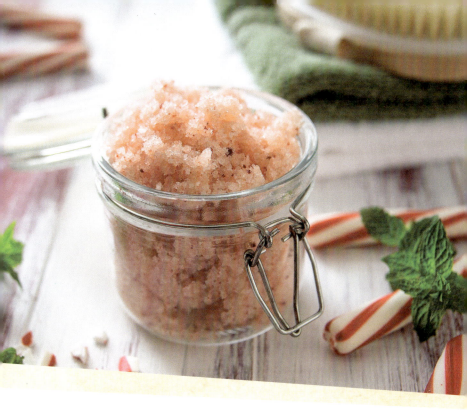

Peppermint Candy

1½ C. pure cane sugar

½ C. coarse sea salt

½ C. olive oil

10 drops peppermint
   essential oil

½ tsp. pure vanilla
   extract

Red food coloring
   (optional)

Follow the basic scrub instructions on page 37. Store in
an airtight container for up to 2 months.

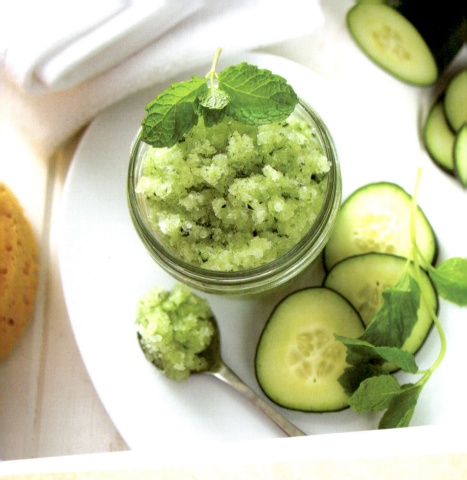

Cucumber Mint

1 small cucumber

¼ C. packed fresh mint
   leaves

1 T. olive oil

1 C. Epsom salt

1 C. coarse sea salt

3 drops peppermint
   essential oil

1. Rinse and roughly chop the cucumber into 1" slices.

2. Puree the cucumber slices, mint, and olive oil in a blender or food processor.

3. In a large bowl, stir together the Epsom salt, sea salt, and cucumber puree.

   Note: depending on the amount of puree, more or less Epsom salt may need to be added to reach the desired consistency.

4. Drop in the essential oil and stir until evenly dispersed throughout the mixture.

5. Transfer the scrub into an airtight container.

6. Store in the refrigerator for up to 3 weeks.

Gifting

Transfer the scrub into a mason jar and cover with coordinating fabric. Fasten a tag to the jar for a decorative touch.

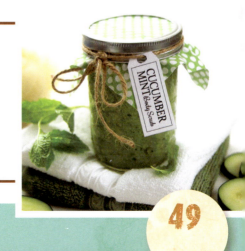

Tub Teas

Common **tub tea** ingredients include:

Epsom Salt is believed to soothe muscle pain.

Salt is full of beneficial minerals that rehydrate and soften skin.

Powdered Milk contains fats and proteins that help hydrate skin and retain moisture.

Oatmeal has anti-inflammatory properties that soothe itchy or irritated skin.

Essential Oils are an easy way to add soothing fragrances to tub teas. They are also known to have many skin and wellness benefits.

Add-ins steep in the hot water and help give tub teas their soothing properties. Since tub teas are strained through a bag or filter, there's no need to limit the amount of add-ins! Dried herbs, flowers, teas, and spices are all great options!

Teabags or Filters are needed to keep the loose tea contained for easy cleanup. Disposable tea filters, reusable muslin bags, metal tea infusers, and homemade cloth bags all work well.

*Follow the basic instructions below when making **tub teas**. Each recipe will make enough tea for approximately 6 baths.*

1. Whisk together the dry ingredients.

2. Add any essential oils or extracts and mix until they're evenly dispersed throughout the mixture.

3. Add any dried flowers, spices, herbs, or teas and gently combine.

4. Store loose tea in an airtight container or prefill teabags for easy use.

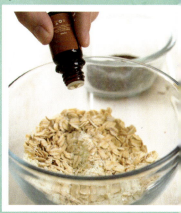

How to use tub teas:

The easiest way to use tub tea is to fill a teabag or filter with 1-2 tablespoons of tub tea and add it to a warm bath. However, if you want to extract the most from your tub teas follow these steps:

1. *Run a warm bath as usual.*

2. *Microwave one cup of water or boil it in a kettle.*

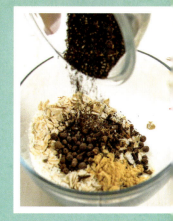

3. *Put the teabag in a mug and cover with one cup of hot water; let steep for one minute.*

4. *Pour the mug of water and the teabag into your bath, but be sure not to get the bath too hot. This process gives the tea a head start on the steeping process without overheating your bath!*

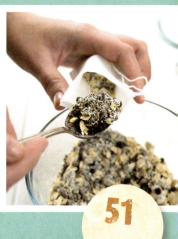

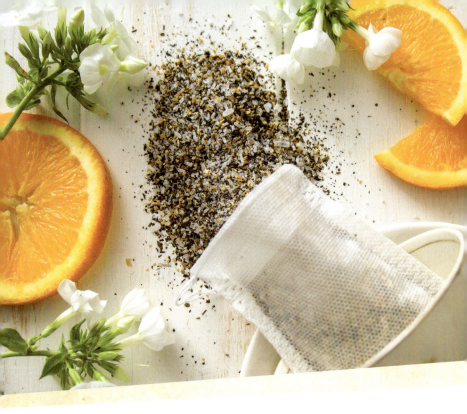

Sweet Jasmine

½ C. Epsom salt

3 drops jasmine
    essential oil

3 drops sweet orange
    essential oil

The contents of
    10 jasmine teabags

¼ C. dried orange peel

Follow the basic tub tea instructions on page 51.

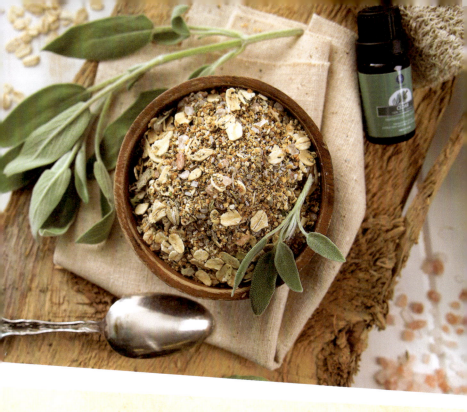

Cedarwood & Sage

¼ C. old-fashioned oats

2 T. Himalayan pink salt

2 T. Epsom salt

15 drops cedar
   essential oil

¼ C. dried leaf sage

¼ C. dried orange peel

The contents of 4 green
   teabags

Follow the basic tub tea instructions on page 51.

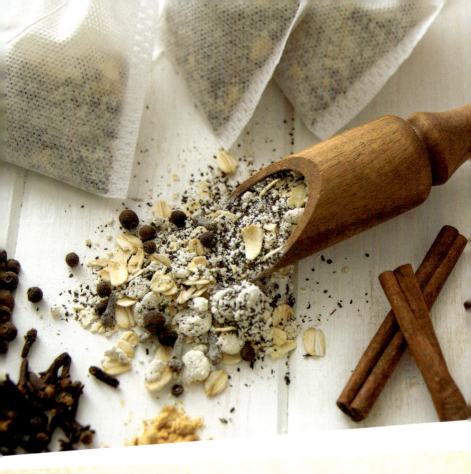

Vanilla Chai

¼ C. powdered milk

¼ C. old-fashioned oats

2 drops cinnamon
 essential oil

½ tsp. pure vanilla extract

The contents of 5 chai
 teabags

2 tsp. whole allspice

2 tsp. whole cloves

1 tsp. ground ginger

1 tsp. ground cinnamon

1. Whisk together the powdered milk and oats.

2. Add the essential oil and extract and mix until they're evenly dispersed throughout the mixture. Be sure to break up any large clumps that may have formed.

3. Cut open the chai teabags and add the contents to the mixture.

4. Add the allspice, cloves, ginger, and cinnamon and gently stir until combined.

5. Store loose tea in an airtight container or prefill teabags for easy use.

Gifting

Easily create your own teabags with scraps of fabric by cutting out small squares, filling the centers with tub tea, and cinching shut with string.

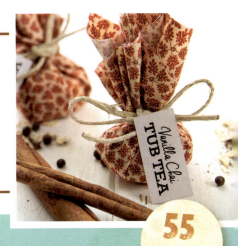

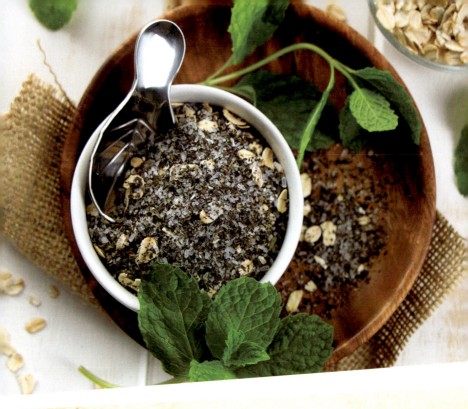

Green Tea Mint

¼ C. Epsom salt

¼ C. old-fashioned oats

4 drops peppermint
essential oil

The contents of 10 green
teabags

¼ C. dried mint

Follow the basic tub tea instructions on page 51.

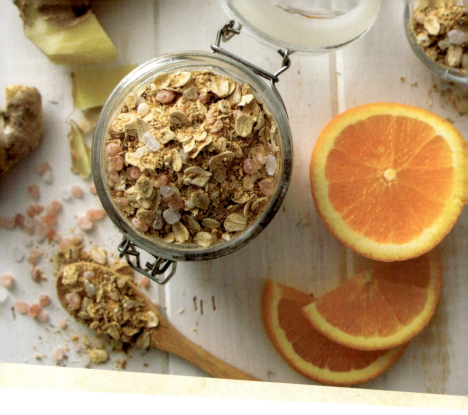

Orange Ginger

2 T. Himalayan pink salt

¼ C. old-fashioned oats

4 drops sweet orange
   essential oil

¼ C. dried orange peel

1 T. ground ginger

The contents of
   4 chamomile teabags

Follow the basic tub tea instructions on page 51.

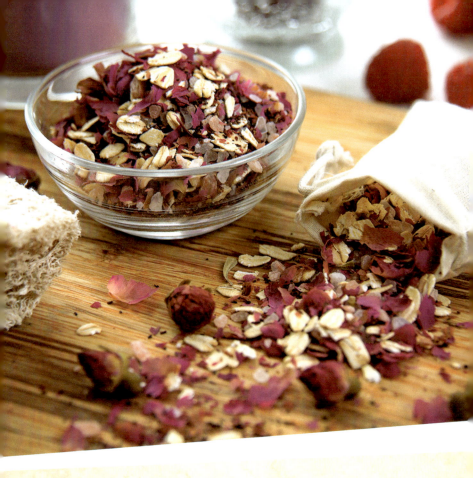

Raspberry Rose

¼ C. old-fashioned oats

¼ C. Himalayan pink salt

3 drops rose essential oil

The contents of 10 raspberry herbal teabags

¼ C. dried rose buds

1. Whisk together the oats and salt.

2. Add the essential oil and mix until evenly dispersed throughout the mixture.

3. Cut open the raspberry teabags and stir the contents into the mixture.

4. Remove the hard, green bases from the rose buds and crush the buds into smaller pieces.

5. Gently stir the crushed rose buds into the tea mixture.

6. Store the loose tea in an airtight container or prefill teabags for easy use.

Gifting

Prefill disposable teabags and bundle them together with twine to create a gift pack. These ready-to-use teabags make for a convenient bath!

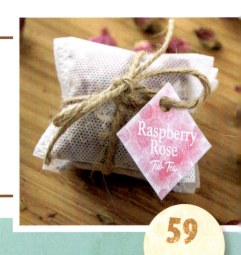

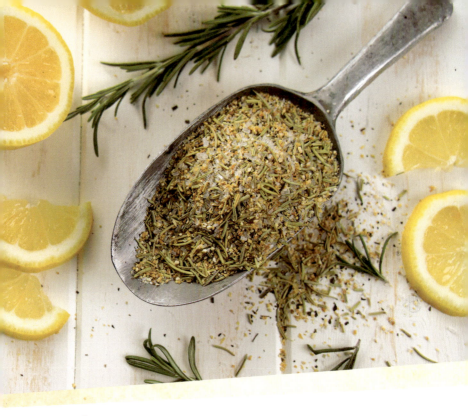

Lemon Rosemary

¼ C. Epsom salt

6 drops lemongrass
    essential oil

3 drops rosemary
    essential oil

¼ C. dried lemon peel

¼ C. dried rosemary

The contents of
    3 chamomile teabags

Follow the basic tub tea instructions on page 51.

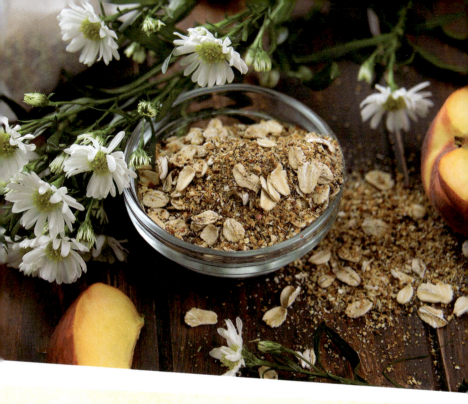

Chamomile Peach

½ C. old-fashioned oats

2 drops chamomile
    essential oil

2 drops sweet orange
    essential oil

The contents of 10 herbal
    peach teabags

The contents of
    5 chamomile teabags

2 T. dried orange peel

1 T. dried lemon peel

Follow the basic tub tea instructions on page 51.

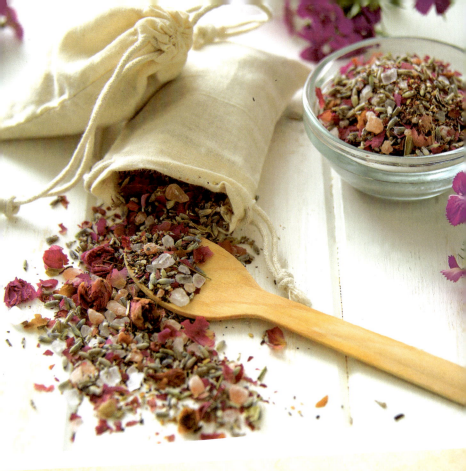

Wildflower

¼ C. Himalayan pink salt

¼ C. dried lavender buds

3 drops lavender
   essential oil

The contents of 8 hibiscus
   teabags

The contents of
   3 chamomile teabags

¼ C. dried rose buds

1. Gently stir together the Himalayan pink salt and lavender buds.

2. Drop in the essential oil and stir until evenly dispersed throughout the mixture.

3. Cut open the hibiscus and chamomile teabags and stir the contents into the mixture.

4. Remove the hard, green bases from the rose buds and crush the buds into smaller pieces.

5. Gently stir the crushed rose buds into the tea mixture.

6. Store the loose tea in an airtight container or prefill teabags for easy use.

Gifting

Fill a small jar with tub tea and include a metal tea infuser. Add a tag to complete the gift!

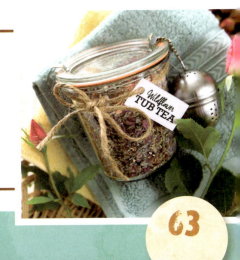

Index

Bath Bombs........................ 4

Candy Cane 12

Double Mint 17

Funfetti................................... 11

Green Tea............................... 16

Lemon Drop............................7

Lovely Lavender 14

Milk & Honey 21

Ocean Breeze 10

Orange Creamsicle 8

Pink Rose 6

Pumpkin Spice Latte........... 18

Warm Woods.......................... 20

Bath Salts........................ 22

Eucalyptus Lavender.......... 25

Gingerbread 28

Lavender Chamomile......... 30

Lemon Thyme 29

Mojito 24

Mountain Air 32

Rose Milk............................... 26

Rosemary Mint..................... 33

Soothing Hot Cocoa........... 34

Body Scrubs.................... 36

Citrus Ginger 46

Coconut Lime 38

Cookie Dough 39

Cucumber Mint.................... 48

Honey Lemon....................... 42

Lavender Oats 43

Lemon Poppy Seed............. 40

Peppermint Candy.............. 47

Spiced Mocha....................... 44

Tub Teas.......................... 50

Cedarwood & Sage 53

Chamomile Peach 61

Green Tea Mint 56

Lemon Rosemary 60

Orange Ginger 57

Raspberry Rose.................... 58

Sweet Jasmine..................... 52

Vanilla Chai 54

Wildflower............................. 62

Gifting Ideas

Bath Bombs 9, 13, 15, 19

Bath Salts 27, 31, 35

Body Scrubs 41, 45, 49

Tub Teas.................55, 59, 63